INTERMITTENT FASTING FOR WOMEN OVER 60

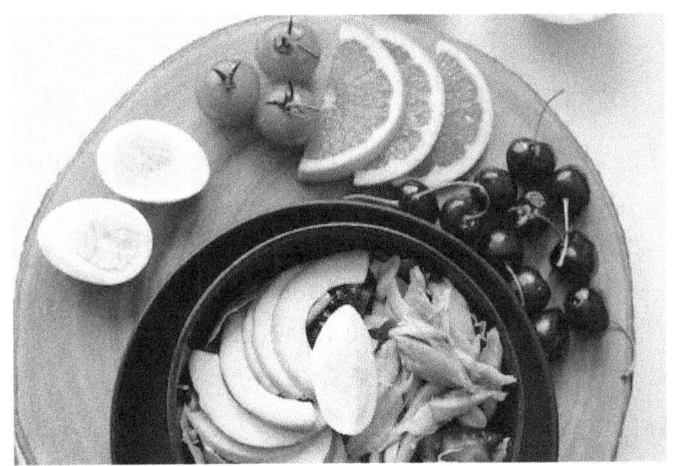

A Comprehensive Guide to Intermittent Fasting for Women - Unlocking Vitality, Wellness, and Longevity with Expert Strategies and Delicious Recipes"

Regina Mery

TABLE OF CONTENTS

CHAPTER 10: THE FINALE CURTAIN CALL

INTRODUCTION

Welcome to "Thriving After 60: A Comprehensive Guide to Intermittent Fasting for Women"!

Are you ready to unlock the secrets to vitality, wellness, and longevity? If you're a woman over 60 looking to rejuvenate your health and embrace a vibrant lifestyle, then this book is your ultimate companion on the journey to wellness.

Intermittent fasting has emerged as a powerful tool for optimizing health and promoting longevity, and its benefits are particularly relevant for women navigating the golden years of life.

In this comprehensive guide, we'll delve into the transformative power of intermittent fasting, offering expert strategies, practical tips, and delicious recipes tailored specifically for women over 60.

CHAPTER 1: THE ART OF FASTING

Unlocking the Rhythms of Intermittent Fasting

Welcome to the gateway of a transformative journey—a journey that reshapes not just your meal times but the very essence of how you approach wellness. We will uncover the essence of intermittent fasting and its remarkable resonance for women gracefully navigating the vibrant shores of their 60s and beyond.

Intermittent fasting isn't a quick fix or a whimsical diet trend; it's an art form—a rhythmic dance with time that taps into the body's innate wisdom. It's about embracing a lifestyle where meals aren't just sustenance but moments of synchronized harmony with your body's natural rhythms.

As we embark on this exploration, we invite you to shed preconceptions and embrace the potential for renewal. Intermittent fasting isn't a rigid discipline; it's a canvas for empowerment, nurturing a relationship with food and well-being that transcends conventional norms.

What is Intermittent Fasting, and How Does It Work?

Intermittent fasting (IF) is an eating pattern that alternates between periods of fasting and eating. It doesn't prescribe specific foods but rather focuses on when to eat. By restricting the time window for eating, IF can help regulate metabolism, promote weight loss, improve insulin sensitivity, and enhance cellular repair processes.

CHAPTER 2: NOURISHING WISDOM FOR SEASONED WOMEN

Discovering the Fountain of Health Beyond 60

The journey into the vibrant years beyond 60 is a journey rich in experiences and the art of nurturing well-being. Intermittent fasting, when tailored to the needs of women in this phase of life, becomes a beacon guiding the quest for health and vitality.

Benefits of Intermittent Fasting

1. Embracing Holistic Wellness

Wellness becomes a holistic pursuit, encompassing not just the physical but also the mental and spiritual aspects of life. Intermittent fasting acts as a companion, encouraging mindful nourishment, fostering resilience, and nurturing a balanced approach to health that transcends mere numbers on a scale.

2. Empowering Weight Management

The concept of weight management evolves into a beautiful relationship between body and nourishment. Intermittent fasting offers a flexible strategy, not just for shedding pounds but for embracing a sustainable and balanced approach to body composition and well-being.

3. Vitality Through Metabolic Health

As the body traverses the years, metabolic health assumes a pivotal role. Intermittent fasting, with its potential to influence metabolic markers, becomes a nurturing ally in supporting overall health, potentially shielding against age-related metabolic concerns.

4. Cognitive Enrichment and Mental Clarity

The treasure of mental acuity and cognitive health gains prominence. Intermittent fasting presents an intriguing avenue for nurturing mental clarity, potentially supporting brain health and offering an empowering approach to preserving cognitive function.

5. Personalized Wellness: Tailoring Health for This Stage

The beauty of intermittent fasting lies in its adaptability. It is not a rigid structure but a versatile tool, uniquely molded to address the specific needs of women over 60. Whether fortifying bone health, navigating hormonal changes, or bolstering immunity, intermittent fasting adapts to empower wellness tailored for this vibrant phase of life.

CHAPTER 3: FASTING STYLES UNVEILED

From Clockwork to Freedom:

Exploring Varied Fasting Schedules

A quote by **Beverly Diehl** states that — **'Everybody is different, and every body is different.**

In the world of health, one size never fits all."

This saying encapsulates the essence of individuality in health pursuits, emphasizing that there isn't a universal solution. It aligns well with the notion that each person's body, wellness journey, including their approach to fasting, is unique and should be tailored to their individual needs and preferences.

Thankfully, when it comes to intermittent fasting, there exists different fasting styles, each offering a unique manner and approach to aligning meals with the body's natural cycles. It's also essential to listen to your body and adjust your fasting schedule as needed. Consulting with a healthcare professional before starting any fasting regimen is recommended, especially for women over 60 or those with underlying health conditions. This chapter unravels different fasting schedules, showcasing the range of options available to women over 60 seeking to embark on an intermittent fasting journey.

They are as follows:

1. Time-Restricted Eating: The Art of Timely Nourishment

Time-Restricted Eating operates on a simple principle—restricting the eating window within specific hours of the day. This approach allows individuals to feast during a predetermined time frame and fast during the remaining hours. It's akin to setting the clock for nourishment, potentially aiding in weight management and improving metabolic health.

Below are some examples of the Time Restricted Eating Method

- **16/8 Method**: This is one of the most common variations of time-restricted feeding. It involves fasting for 16 hours each day and restricting your eating window to 8 hours. For example, one might eat from 12:00 PM to 8:00 PM and fast from 8:00 PM to 12:00 PM the next day.

- **14/10 Method:** Similar to the 16/8 method, the 14/10 method involves fasting for 14 hours and eating within a 10-hour window. For instance, one might eat from 10:00 AM to 8:00 PM and fast from 8:00 PM to 10:00 AM the next day.

- **12/12 Method:** This method is less restrictive and involves fasting for 12 hours and eating within a 12-hour window. For example, one might eat from 8:00 AM to 8:00 PM and fast from 8:00 PM to 8:00 AM the next day.

- **18/6 Method**: For those who prefer a longer fasting period, the 18/6 method involves fasting for 18 hours and consuming all meals within a 6-hour window. For example, one might eat from 2:00 PM to 8:00 PM and fast from 8:00 PM to 2:00 PM the next day.

- **20/4 Method (Warrior Diet):** This method is more extreme, with a fasting period of 20 hours and an eating window of 4 hours. The Warrior Diet typically involves consuming one large meal in the evening. For example, one might eat from 4:00 PM to 8:00 PM and fast from 8:00 PM to 4:00 PM the next day.

These are just a few examples of time-restricted feeding methods..

2. Alternate-Day Fasting: Embracing Intermittent Abstinence

Alternate-Day Fasting offers a pattern where individuals alternate between days of normal eating and days of reduced calorie intake. This approach introduces cycles of feast and fast, potentially leading to weight loss and metabolic improvements. However, it requires adaptability, as some may find the alternating days challenging to integrate into their routine.

3. The 5:2 Method: A Blend of Moderation and Intermittence

The 5:2 Method involves eating normally for five days a week and limiting calorie intake on two non-consecutive days. This approach intertwines regular eating with intermittent fasting, offering a balance between moderation and calorie restriction. It may aid in weight management and metabolic health while allowing for flexibility on non-fasting days.

4. Modified Fasting Schedules: Tailoring Fasting to Individual Needs

Amidst the structured approaches, Modified Fasting Schedules offer flexibility. This style allows individuals to personalize fasting periods based on their preferences and lifestyle. It's an adaptable approach, empowering individuals to adjust fasting days to suit their routine, potentially making intermittent fasting more sustainable and integrated into daily life.

5. Exploring Freedom in Fasting: Adapting to Individual Lifestyles

Intermittent fasting isn't merely about adhering to strict schedules but finding a rhythm that aligns seamlessly with individual lifestyles. Whether it's aligning fasting with social commitments, exercise routines, or work schedules, the essence lies in discovering a fasting style that resonates personally and feels sustainable in the long run.

The key is to choose a fasting window that fits your lifestyle, preferences, and health goals, while ensuring that you still meet your nutritional needs during your eating window

CHAPTER 4: EMBARKING ON THE FASTING JOURNEY

Safely Setting Sail and Choosing Your Course

Embarking on an intermittent fasting journey requires thoughtful consideration and preparation, especially for women navigating the vibrant chapter of their 60s and beyond. This phase is akin to setting sail on uncharted waters, demanding a careful approach to ensure a safe and fulfilling voyage towards improved health and well-being.

Understanding Your Body's Signals

Before hoisting the sails, it's crucial to assess your readiness. Take stock of your health conditions, listen to your body's signals, and consider any potential impacts of fasting. This initial understanding allows for a more informed and safe commencement of your fasting adventure.

Charting Your Fasting Course

Navigating the sea of fasting styles is the next step. Explore the array of options as discussed in the previous chapter—Time-Restricted Eating, Alternate-Day Fasting, 5:2 Method, and Modified Fasting Schedules. Delve into their nuances, weighing their benefits and challenges against your lifestyle and health aspirations to chart a fasting course that resonates with your individual journey.

Preparing the Vessel for Your Journey

Prepare for the voyage by easing into fasting gradually. Make gentle adjustments in meal timings, experiment with shorter fasting windows, and adapt meal compositions. These gradual shifts serve as a compass, guiding you into the fasting rhythm with reduced turbulence.

Anticipating and Managing Challenges

Rough waters are inevitable. Anticipate challenges such as managing hunger, navigating social situations, and dealing with initial discomforts. Equip yourself with strategies and tools to weather these challenges, ensuring a smoother and more confident sailing into intermittent fasting.

Monitoring Progress and Adjusting Your Course

As you journey forward, keep a watchful eye on your progress. Monitor your health markers, energy levels, and overall well-being. Understand your body's unique responses to fasting, allowing you to adjust and fine-tune your fasting routine as needed, ensuring a course that aligns harmoniously with your well-being.

Cultivating Long-Term Sustainability

View intermittent fasting not merely as a short-term endeavor but as a sustainable lifestyle choice. Integrate fasting seamlessly into your daily routine, nurturing a mindset that fosters resilience, supporting long-term health, and vitality throughout your journey.

CHAPTER 5: SECRETS TO THRIVING

Real-Life Lessons From the Journey

In a quaint neighborhood lived Sarah, a vibrant woman in her 60s. Sarah's journey into intermittent fasting was a realistic adventure, not just a quest for health but a pursuit of vitality that resonated deeply with her daily life.

Sarah's mornings once brimmed with routines—coffee with friends, morning walks, and cherishing time with her grandchildren. But she longed for a shift, a new energy that could infuse more vibrancy into her days.

With cautious curiosity, Sarah embarked on an intermittent fasting journey, seeking a lifestyle change that wouldn't compromise her cherished moments but rather enhance them.

Through trial and error, Sarah discovered a few secrets to thriving with intermittent fasting for women over 60:

Listening to Your Body: Sarah quickly learned the importance of listening to her body. Fasting wasn't just about timing meals but tuning into hunger cues, ensuring she felt nourished and energized, not deprived.

Flexibility and Adaptability: Sarah found her rhythm in the flexibility of Modified Fasting Schedules. This style allowed her to adapt fasting periods to accommodate family gatherings and social outings, empowering her to enjoy these moments while honoring her fasting routine.

Mindful Nutrition: Embracing nutritious meals became Sarah's mantra. She focused on wholesome, nutrient-rich foods during her eating windows, amplifying the benefits of fasting by nourishing her body with quality nutrition.

Support and Community: Sarah discovered strength in community. Sharing experiences and tips with like-minded individuals provided encouragement, motivation, and valuable insights that enriched her fasting journey.

Patience and Persistence: Above all, Sarah learned patience and persistence. Embracing intermittent fasting wasn't an overnight transformation but a gradual evolution. She persevered through initial challenges, knowing that consistency and patience were keys to long-term success.

Your keys to success

Repeat after me **"Nourishment, Hydration, and Movement! "**

Embarking on an intermittent fasting journey requires careful attention to nourishment, hydration, and movement to ensure success and well-being. By prioritizing these key elements, individuals can optimize their fasting experience and reap the benefits of improved health and vitality. Let's explore how nourishment, hydration, and movement serve as essential pillars of success in intermittent fasting.

Nourishment:

Nourishing your body with nutrient-dense foods during your eating window is essential for sustaining energy levels, supporting overall health, and maximizing the benefits of intermittent fasting. Focus on incorporating a variety of whole foods, including fruits, vegetables, lean proteins, whole grains, and healthy fats, to provide essential vitamins, minerals, and antioxidants.

Choose complex carbohydrates such as whole grains, legumes, and starchy vegetables to provide sustained energy and fiber for digestive health.

Prioritize lean proteins like poultry, fish, tofu, and legumes to support muscle repair and growth.

Include healthy fats from sources such as nuts, seeds, avocado, and olive oil to promote satiety and support brain health.

Limit processed foods, refined sugars, and unhealthy fats, which can lead to energy crashes and disrupt metabolic health.

Hydration:

Staying hydrated is crucial during intermittent fasting to support bodily functions, regulate appetite, and prevent dehydration. Aim to drink plenty of water throughout the day, especially during your eating window, to maintain hydration levels and support overall well-being.

Start your day with a glass of water to rehydrate after fasting overnight and kickstart your metabolism.

Keep a water bottle with you throughout the day as a reminder to drink regularly.

Hydrate with herbal teas, infused water, or electrolyte-rich beverages during fasting periods to support hydration and curb hunger.

Monitor your urine color and hydration status to ensure adequate fluid intake, aiming for pale yellow urine as a sign of proper hydration.

Movement:

Incorporating regular physical activity into your routine complements intermittent fasting by supporting metabolism, preserving lean muscle mass, and enhancing overall health and well-being. Find activities that you enjoy and can sustainably incorporate into your lifestyle, whether it's walking, cycling, yoga, or strength training.

Schedule workouts during your eating window to fuel your body with energy and nutrients for optimal performance.

Incorporate movement throughout the day by taking short walks, stretching breaks, or engaging in household chores to avoid prolonged periods of sitting.

Listen to your body and adjust the intensity and duration of your workouts based on how you feel during fasting periods.

Prioritize consistency over intensity, aiming for regular physical activity that you can maintain over time to support long-term health and wellness.

CHAPTER 6: TAMING THE HUNGER DRAGON

Conquering Cravings, Breaking Barriers, and Social Grace

Conquering Cravings:

Focus on Nutrient-Dense Foods: During eating windows, prioritize whole, nutrient-dense foods like fruits, vegetables, lean proteins, and healthy fats. These foods can help keep you fuller for longer and reduce cravings for processed snacks.

Stay Hydrated: Dehydration can often be mistaken for hunger. Drink plenty of water throughout the day, especially during fasting periods, to curb cravings and support overall health.

Incorporate Fiber: Fiber-rich foods like whole grains, legumes, and vegetables can aid in digestion, promote satiety, and stabilize blood sugar levels, reducing the likelihood of cravings.

Mindful Eating: Pay attention to hunger cues and practice mindful eating during meal times. Chew slowly, savor each bite, and listen to your body's signals of fullness.

Breaking Barriers:

Start Slow: If you're new to intermittent fasting, ease into it gradually by gradually increasing fasting periods over time. This approach can help your body adjust and reduce the likelihood of feeling overwhelmed.

Listen to Your Body: Pay attention to how your body responds to fasting. If you experience dizziness, fatigue, or other adverse effects, consider adjusting your fasting schedule or consulting with a healthcare professional.

Customize Your Approach: Like already established before, Intermittent fasting is not one-size-fits-all. Experiment with different fasting protocols to find what works best for your body and lifestyle.

Prioritize Self-Care: Incorporate stress-reducing activities like yoga, meditation, or leisurely walks into your routine to support overall well-being during fasting periods.

Social Grace:

Communicate Effectively: Inform friends, family, and social circles about your intermittent fasting journey. Educate them on your chosen fasting schedule and any dietary restrictions you may have to help avoid awkward situations.

Plan Ahead: When attending social gatherings or dining out, plan ahead by bringing your own snacks or suggesting restaurants that offer fasting-friendly options.

Focus on Socialization: Shift the focus of social gatherings from food to meaningful conversations and activities. Engage in hobbies, games, or walks with friends and loved ones to maintain social connections without solely relying on food.

Be Flexible: While it's essential to stick to your fasting schedule, allow yourself flexibility on occasion. Life happens, and it's okay to adjust your fasting window to accommodate special events or social occasions.

Chapter 7: ADJUSTING YOUR FASTING WINDOW

Adjusting your fasting window refers to modifying the duration of time you abstain from consuming calories during intermittent fasting. The fasting window typically involves a period where you refrain from eating, followed by a window where you consume meals and calories. This adjustment can be made to better suit your lifestyle, preferences, or to address any specific health concerns.

Let's consider a realistic example to illustrate this concept:

Original Fasting Window: Initially, you decide to follow a 16/8 intermittent fasting schedule, where you fast for 16 hours and have an 8-hour eating window. For instance, you might choose to eat from 12:00 PM to 8:00 PM and fast from 8:00 PM to 12:00 PM the next day.

Reason for Adjustment: You find that you're experiencing intense hunger or cravings late in the evening, making it challenging to adhere to your fasting schedule. This can lead to overeating or consuming unhealthy foods during your eating window, which may undermine your overall health goals.

Adjusted Fasting Window: To address this issue, you decide to adjust your fasting window to include more of your waking hours, when distractions and activities can help keep hunger at bay.

Adjusted Fasting Window Scenario

Old Fasting Window: Fasting from 8:00 PM to 12:00 PM (16/8 schedule)

New Fasting Window: Fasting from 6:00 PM to 10:00 AM (16/8 schedule)

With this adjustment:

You finish your last meal earlier in the evening, around 6:00 PM, reducing the likelihood of experiencing intense hunger or cravings before bedtime.

You wake up with a shorter fasting period remaining, making it psychologically easier to continue fasting until your eating window begins at 10:00 AM.

By making this adjustment, you can potentially reduce the temptation to overeat or consume unhealthy foods during the fasting period, improving your ability to stick to your intermittent fasting regimen and achieve your health goals.

CHAPTER 8: CULINARY SYMPHONY: 20 RECIPES FOR FASTING FEASTS

Quinoa breakfast bowl

Ingredients:

1 cup quinoa

Mixed berries (strawberries, blueberries, raspberries)

Handful of nuts (almonds, walnuts)

Honey (optional)

Procedure:

Cook quinoa according to package instructions.

Serve in a bowl, topped with mixed berries, nuts, and a drizzle of honey if desired.

Suitable for: Breakfast

2. Avocado and egg salad

Ingredients:

2 avocados

4 boiled eggs

Mixed greens

Vinaigrette (olive oil, vinegar, mustard)

Procedure:

Slice avocados and eggs.

Arrange over a bed of mixed greens.

Dress with vinaigrette made with olive oil, vinegar, and mustard.

Suitable for: Lunch

3. Roasted Vegetable soup

Ingredients:

3 carrots

2 bell peppers

4 tomatoes

Herbs (rosemary, thyme)

Procedure:

Chop vegetables and toss with herbs.

Roast in the oven until tender.

Blend roasted vegetables with water/vegetable broth until smooth.

Suitable for: Lunch or Dinner

4. Grilled chicken with Asparagus

Ingredients:

4 chicken breasts

1 bunch asparagus

Seasoning (salt, pepper, garlic powder)

Procedure:

Season chicken and asparagus.

Grill until chicken is cooked through and asparagus is tender.

Suitable for: Dinner

5. Chia seed pudding

Ingredients:

1/2 cup chia seeds

2 cups almond milk

Fruits (berries, mango)

Nuts (almonds, pistachios)

Procedure:

Mix chia seeds with almond milk.

Refrigerate overnight.

Top with fruits and nuts before serving.

Suitable for: Breakfast or Snack

6. Cauliflower rice stir-fry

Ingredients:

1 head cauliflower

Assorted veggies (bell peppers, broccoli, carrots)

Tofu/Chicken/Shrimp (optional)

Soy sauce, garlic, ginger (for seasoning)

Procedure:

Pulse cauliflower in a food processor to rice-like texture.

Stir-fry with veggies and protein of choice.

Season with soy sauce, garlic, and ginger.

Suitable for: Lunch or Dinner

7. Mediterranean Salad

Ingredients:

Mixed greens

Cucumber, tomatoes, olives

Feta cheese

Lemon-olive oil dressing

Procedure:

Toss together mixed greens, chopped vegetables, olives, and feta cheese.

Dress with lemon-olive oil dressing.

Suitable for: Lunch or Dinner

8. Salmon with Roasted Vegetables

Ingredients:

Salmon fillets

Broccoli, Brussels sprouts, sweet potatoes

Olive oil, herbs

Procedure:

Roast salmon and vegetables with olive oil and herbs until cooked.

Suitable for: Dinner

9. Greek Yogurt Parfait

Ingredients:

Greek yogurt

Berries, granola

Honey (optional)

Procedure:

Layer yogurt, berries, granola, and honey in a glass.

Suitable for: Breakfast or Snack

10. Zucchini Noodles with Pesto

Ingredients:

Zucchini

Pesto sauce

Cherry tomatoes

Procedure:

Spiralize zucchini.

Toss with pesto sauce and cherry tomatoes.

Suitable for: Lunch or Dinner

11. Turkey Lettuce Wraps

Ingredients:

1 lb ground turkey

Lettuce leaves (1 head)

2 tablespoons soy sauce

1 teaspoon minced ginger

2 cloves garlic, minced

1 cup diced water chestnuts

1 bell pepper, diced

1 carrot, grated

Procedure:

Cook ground turkey with soy sauce, ginger, and garlic until browned.

Add water chestnuts, bell pepper, and grated carrot, cook until veggies soften.

Spoon the mixture onto lettuce leaves, wrap, and enjoy.

Suitable for: Lunch or Dinner

12. Eggplant Caponata

Ingredients:

1 large eggplant, diced

3 tomatoes, diced

2 tablespoons capers

1/4 cup sliced olives

3 tablespoons olive oil

2 tablespoons balsamic vinegar

Procedure:

Sauté diced eggplant and tomatoes in olive oil until softened.

Add capers, sliced olives, and balsamic vinegar, simmer for flavors to meld.

Suitable for: Lunch or Dinner

13. Black Bean Salad

Ingredients:

2 cups black beans (canned, drained and rinsed)

1 cup corn kernels

1 bell pepper, diced

1/2 red onion, finely chopped

Lime-cilantro dressing (2 tablespoons lime juice, 1/4 cup chopped cilantro, 2 tablespoons olive oil)

Procedure:

Mix black beans, corn, diced bell pepper, and finely chopped red onion.

Dress with lime-cilantro dressing.

Suitable for: Lunch or Dinner

14. Tuna Stuffed Bell Peppers

Ingredients:

4 bell peppers

2 cans tuna, drained

1 cup cooked quinoa

1 teaspoon paprika

1 teaspoon cumin

Procedure:

Mix drained tuna, cooked quinoa, paprika, and cumin.

Stuff bell peppers, bake until peppers are tender.

Suitable for: Lunch or Dinner

15. Cucumber and Radish Salad

Ingredients:

2 cucumbers

1 cup radishes

2 tablespoons lemon juice

2 tablespoons chopped dill

Procedure:

Slice cucumbers and radishes thinly.

Toss with lemon juice and chopped dill.

Suitable for: Lunch or Dinner

16. Shrimp Stir-Fry with Broccoli

Ingredients:

1 lb shrimp, peeled and deveined

2 cups broccoli florets

1 bell pepper, sliced

2 cloves garlic, minced

2 tablespoons soy sauce

1 teaspoon sesame oil

Procedure:

Stir-fry shrimp until pink, then set aside.

Stir-fry broccoli, bell pepper, and garlic until tender-crisp.

Add cooked shrimp back to the pan, stir in soy sauce and sesame oil.

Suitable for: Lunch or Dinner

17. Cottage Cheese and Fruit Bowl

Ingredients:

2 cups cottage cheese

Assorted fruits (berries, mango, kiwi)

Nuts (almonds, pistachios)

Honey (optional)

Procedure:

Spoon cottage cheese into a bowl.

Top with assorted fruits and nuts. Drizzle with honey if desired.

18. Tofu and Veggie Skewers

Ingredients:

1 block tofu, cubed

Assorted veggies (bell peppers, zucchini, mushrooms)

Marinade (soy sauce, garlic, ginger)

Procedure:

Marinate tofu cubes and veggies in the marinade.

Thread onto skewers and grill until lightly charred.

Suitable for: Lunch or Dinner

19. Cabbage and Carrot Slaw

Ingredients:

4 cups shredded cabbage

1 cup shredded carrots

Dressing (2 tablespoons olive oil, 2 tablespoons apple cider vinegar, 1 teaspoon honey)

Procedure:

Mix shredded cabbage and carrots in a bowl.

Toss with the dressing until well combined.

Suitable for: Lunch or Dinner

20. Baked Apples with Cinnamon

Ingredients:

4 apples, cored and halved

Cinnamon

Honey (optional)

Procedure:

Place apple halves on a baking dish, sprinkle with cinnamon.

Drizzle with honey if desired.

Bake until apples are tender.

Suitable for: Dessert or Snack

NOTE: *Adjustments can be made based on personal preferences and dietary needs.*

CHAPTER 9: QUEST FOR CLARITY:

FAQs Explored

Is Intermittent Fasting Suitable for Everyone? While intermittent fasting can offer various health benefits, it may not be suitable for everyone. Individuals with certain medical conditions, pregnant or breastfeeding women, those with a history of eating disorders, or those with specific nutrient requirements should consult with a healthcare professional before starting intermittent fasting.

Can Intermittent Fasting Help with Weight Loss? Intermittent fasting can aid weight loss by creating a calorie deficit and promoting fat burning. Additionally, it may help regulate hormones related to appetite and metabolism. However, sustainable weight loss also depends on overall dietary choices, portion control, and regular physical activity.

Is Intermittent Fasting Safe for Women Over 60? Intermittent fasting can be safe for women over 60, but it's essential to approach it cautiously and consider individual health circumstances. Consulting with a healthcare professional is crucial to ensure that intermittent fasting is suitable and tailored to specific needs and goals.

What are the potential benefits of intermittent fasting for women over 60? Intermittent fasting may offer various benefits for women over 60, including improved metabolic health, weight management, increased insulin sensitivity, enhanced cellular repair processes, and potential cognitive benefits. However, individual responses may vary, and consulting with a healthcare provider is advisable.

Are there any special considerations or precautions for women over 60 who want to try intermittent fasting? Women over 60 should consider factors such as medications, existing health conditions, nutritional needs, and hormonal changes when embarking on intermittent fasting. It's important to listen to your body, start gradually, stay hydrated, and monitor energy levels and overall well-being. Consulting with a healthcare professional before starting intermittent fasting is crucial, especially for those with underlying health concerns.

Can intermittent fasting help with age-related health concerns in women over 60?
Intermittent fasting may offer potential benefits for age-related health concerns in women over 60, such as reducing inflammation, improving cardiovascular health, enhancing insulin sensitivity, and supporting cognitive function. However, more research is still on going to fully understand the effects of intermittent fasting on specific age-related health conditions. Consulting with a healthcare professional can provide personalized guidance and recommendations based on individual health needs and goals

CHAPTER 12: THE FINALE CURTAIN CALL

As we bid farewell through this chapter, let us carry forward the knowledge gained and the lessons learned, knowing that the journey towards optimal health and vitality is a lifelong pursuit. May these insights you've gained from this book serve as a beacon of guidance and inspiration as you continue on your path, and may you embrace each day with renewed energy, resilience, and joy.

Remember, intermittent fasting is not just about restricting food; it's about nourishing the body, nurturing the spirit, and honoring the wisdom that comes with age. With mindfulness, patience, and a spirit of adventure, may you continue to thrive and flourish in the years to come.

Enjoy your Journey into intermittent fasting, Dearest Reader!

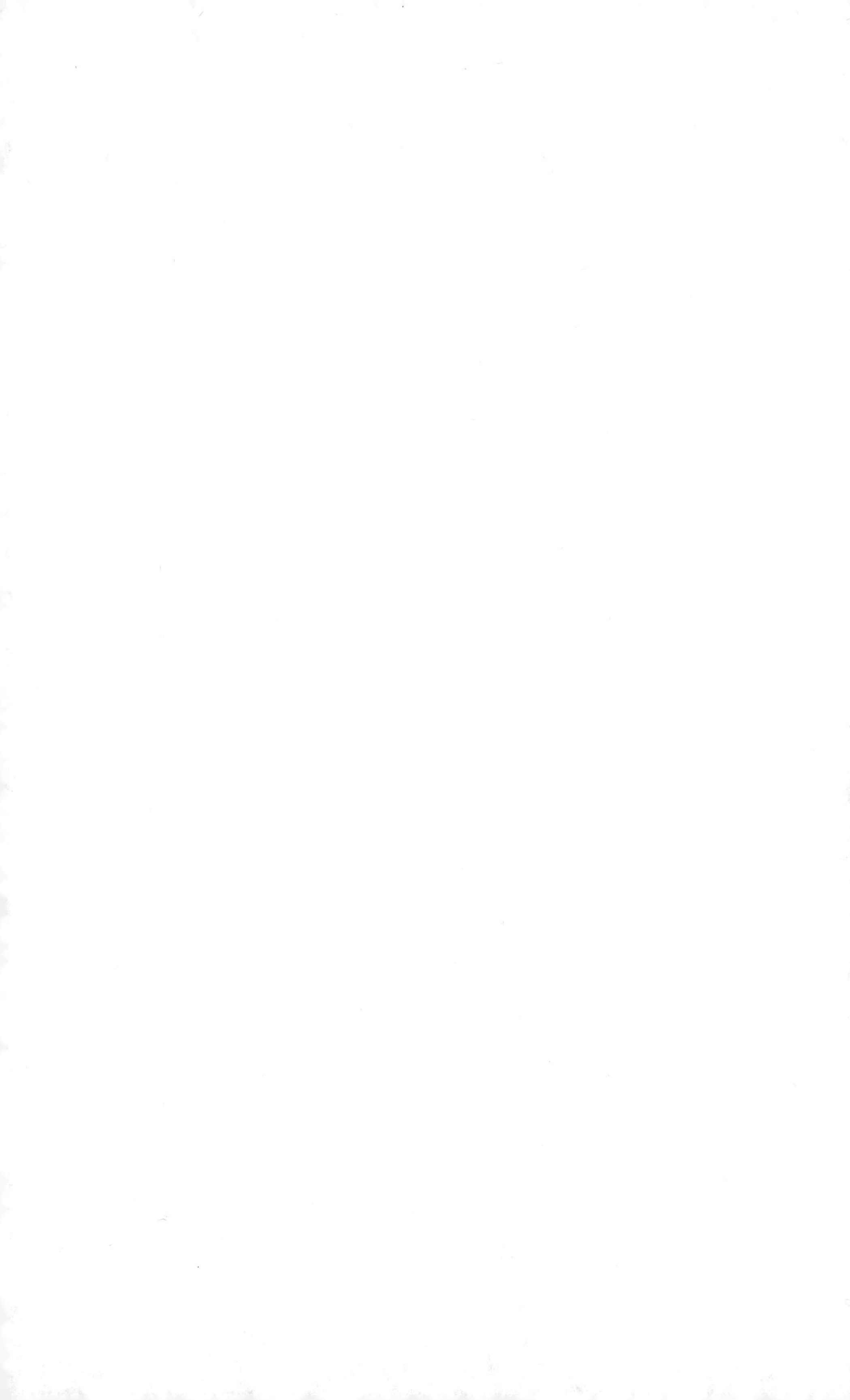

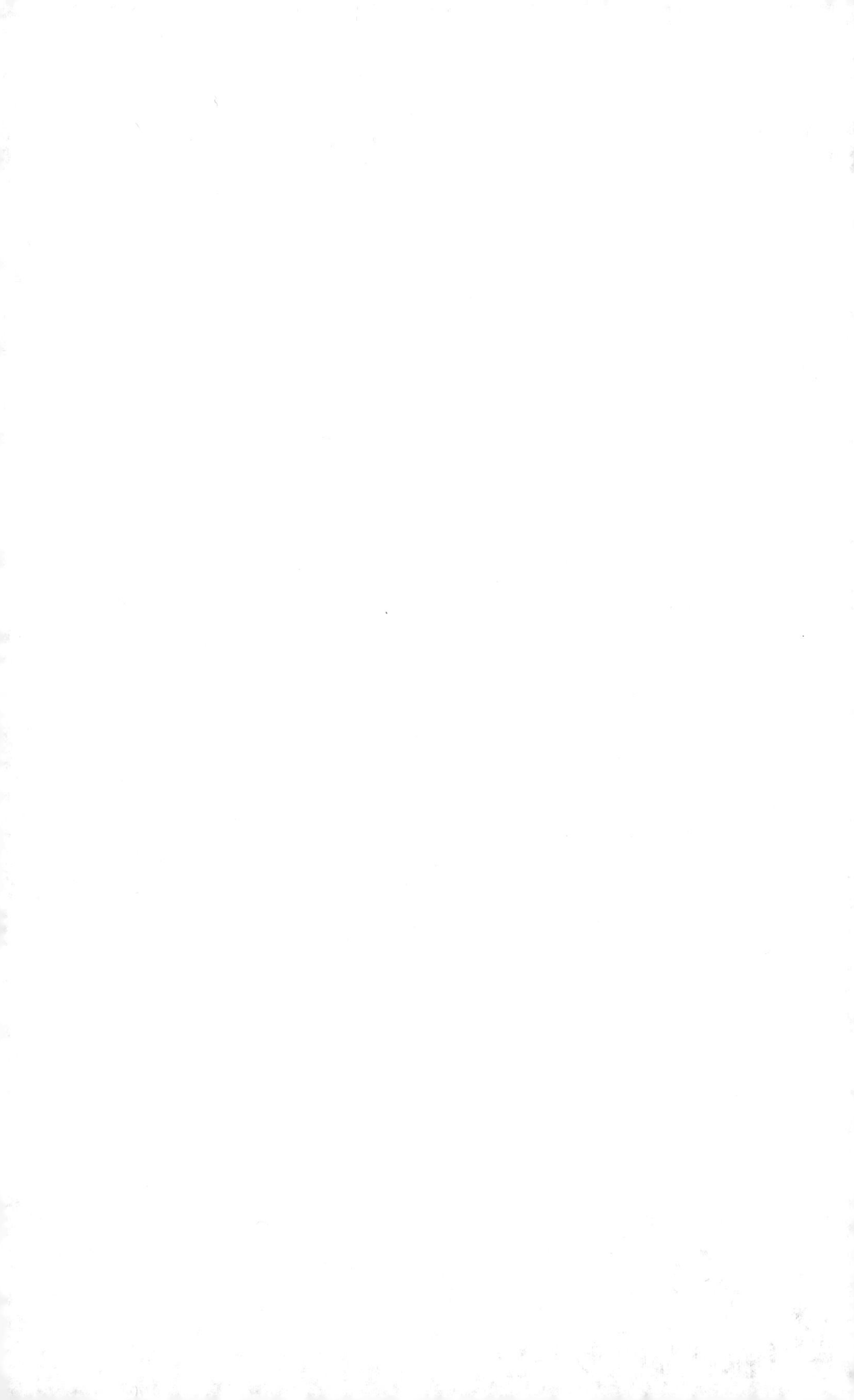